TLP Physical

Health Training Manual

TERRY MILLER

Requests for information or orders contact:
Miller Tribe Publishing, 651 Sunflower Ave, Santa Ana, CA 92707 or 714.546.8911

This book is designed to provide information and motivation to the reader. Every effort has been made to ensure the information in this book is accurate. The author and publisher do not assume and hereby disclaim any liability to any party for any loss, damage, or disruption caused by errors or omissions, whether such errors or omissions result from negligence, accident, or any other cause.

This book is not intended as a substitute for the medical advice of physicians. The reader should regularly consult a physician in matters relating to his/her health and particularly with respect to any symptoms that may require diagnosis or medical attention.

The information in this book is meant to supplement, not replace, proper fitness training. The author and publisher advise readers to take full responsibility for their safety and know their limits. Before practicing the skills described in this book, be sure that your equipment is well maintained, and do not take risks beyond your level of experience, aptitude, training, and comfort level.

Neither the publisher nor author shall be liable for any physical, psychological, emotional, financial, or other damages, including, but not limited to, special, incidental, consequential or other damages.

TotalLifePursuit.org

First edition: March 2019

ISBN: 978-0-9912579-1-1

TABLE OF CONTENTS

Introduction

Welcome to Total Life Pursuit Physical Health Training! Welcome to your next level of productivity! You have decided to become a *healthy* champion in life!

During these next six weeks you will be accelerating towards living beyond how you previously lived. There is no way to become an extraordinary person if you keep doing the same ol' ordinary things. This course is designed to stretch you, empower you and take you to new levels in physical health. You get to choose those levels. It is your life and you have your own starting place. You will be cheered on to complete your training, however, I am hoping that you go far beyond the minimum requirements of this course, and keep it going long after these next six weeks.

We all want remarkable health. After all, who wants to be sick? Who wants to be limited in what we can do with our bodies? We want to live the remarkable life that Jesus came to give. We want it to last our entire lives. During this course of training you will not only learn things you didn't know, but you will be refreshed again by things you had left on the shelf and you will have an opportunity for God to move you to your next level of physical health. You will set your own goals and watch yourself attain them as we give you keys to a healthier physical life with our very practical approach.

The Integrated Life

An aquifer is an underground water table. A spring is where the underground water meets the ground's surface. These often flow into a river along with other tributaries that make up the river. The river runs into a lake, sea or ocean as well as seeping back into the earth to replenish the aquifers. This along with evaporation and condensation brings the cycle of watering the earth and provides water for plants, animals and people. This is a life cycle of this planet and it is a picture of our wholistic or integrated life.

We will be concentrating on improving the river of physical health for the next six weeks. This river of health is fed by the tributaries of spiritual life, mental life, emotional life, relational life and even your financial life. They all add to the river of health. When you have water in one of the tributaries that isn't good, your river will be affected. In the book Emotionally Healthy Spirituality, Peter Scazzero puts forth the idea that your spiritual maturity is in direct correlation to your emotional maturity. In other words, until you grow up emotionally, you can't grow up spiritually beyond a certain point. We cannot, as the integrated people that God has created us to be, disconnect or stop growing in one area of life and expect to reach our peak in another.

For the Christ follower, this means that unless God is invited into your physical life, it will suffer. Think about it for a minute. If the physical doesn't matter then we should be able to do anything physical and it would not impact other areas of our life. Drunkenness, extra-marital sex and a host of other physical things do affect us, as does eating and sleeping. What you eat affects your brain chemistry, which is obviously important to how you think and process the world around you. Our physical life matters to us as it matters to God. It is with this premise that the subject of physical health belongs in the church and requires the effort of discipleship (training), both personal and corporate, to be done and done well.

"Beloved, I pray that you may prosper in all things and be in health, just as your soul prospers."

— *3 John 2 (NKJV)*

We all care about health because God wants us to prosper and "be in health" even as our soul prospers. Just like Papa God wants us to have great marriages, He wants us to have great health. We were given one body; it is His temple and we must nurture, support, and take care of it. This honors Papa God and benefits us. Why? Because Papa God wants US to have the most enjoyable, pleasurable, prosperous life that we can have here on Earth! That doesn't mean our lives will be trouble or pain free. It means that our lives are the best possible for our particular situation. One of the key components of that life is maintaining great health. Health is one of the highest riches. Without health, you cannot enjoy the things God gives you – wealth, relationships, adventures, your mind...everything. Without health, you cannot live out all of the very things God has created for you to do!

Our bodies are so wonderfully made that when we tell them to, they will change. They will get stronger, faster, more stable, and more agile as we exercise and we think properly. Becoming more fit, or losing weight, for some, is just part of the equation to physical health. There is so much more to taking care of our bodies, and much of it is enjoyable!

Our immune systems were created and designed to keep us healthy and to help us recover quickly from every virus and bacteria. Our bodies were designed to burn fat and resist decay. In fact, 80% of what we call aging is actually decaying which is mostly optional. We are able to add years to our life and add quality to our years through proper care and exercise according to God's plan. We can, through our choices, reduce our chances of major disease or maladies up to 80%! Then you add in the power of the Holy Spirit...and you can see where this is going!

With your health in place, you'll be more able to enjoy your time on this Earth. You will become more in tune with God's creation, your body – His temple. You will learn how to fuel, strengthen, and take care of it so that your days are filled with energy and vitality. During the next six weeks, you will get practical tools, knowledge and wisdom to apply to your life in the major area of physical health. You will also have the opportunity to get a glimpse into how other areas of life intersect with your physical health. By focusing mainly on this sole area, you may improve your physical health little by little or by leaps and bounds. The one thing I know for sure is that when we put considerable focus and effort into something, we have a far greater chance of improvement.

You are a champion (a person who has dominion) and not a victim in any way, shape, or form! God has given you authority, power, strength, wisdom and perseverance to be "more than conquerors" (Romans 8:37) of any mountain or valley that is before you. God is for you and is more than your helper, He is the shaper and builder of the "temple" that He purchased – that's YOU! As you abandon yourself to Him and listen to His heart for you, He will take you to new heights!

Enjoy the journey,

Terry

NOTE: This manual is written in context of the full TLP Life Manual. At times you may think you are missing some information or concepts that aren't fully explained here in this Physical manual. Please refer to the full TLP Life Manual for a more complete understanding. The above introduction has been added, along with the last section which is a short theology of the body. I have also added scripture references and journal pages at the end of this workbook for your daily reading and meditation. I encourage you to look up the references and write about them daily in addition to what you normally do on a daily basis.

Physical Life

I know what you're expecting in this chapter. Diet and exercise. After all, those are two of the top three New Year's resolutions. Those two things are talked about more than anything else when it comes to physical health. The marketing of every diet known to mankind, whether it be the Grapefruit Diet, Atkins, DASH, Whole 30, Warrior, South Beach, or eating systems like Weight Watchers, Nutrisystem or Jenny Craig, or the popular Paleo, Keto, Vegan or Vegetarian eating lifestyles, we are bombarded with diets that all claim to get us healthier and thinner.

So what works? In my upcoming book about health made simple I will help all of us discern the voluminous information about diets. This manual centers on physical health in a more holistic way. What if I told you that sunlight was vitally important to health? What if I purported that laughing and enjoyment is a must for a healthy body? You may say that experts claim health is 80% diet. If you are eating and drinking (intake) wonderful things but you are sedentary, depressed, lonely, live in a dungeon with no fresh air or sunlight, sleep horribly, have a high stress job and you work seven days a week...well, you get the point. Intake is important, but to focus solely on intake because experts claim 80% of your health depends on it, is missing the big picture. Health is a state of being that is attained by more than eating organic greens.

Having said that, this manual will focus on eating and movement, but will not neglect the other very important factors of physical health and fitness. There are other factors such as stress, forgiveness and thinking that I will not go into deeply here as they will be addressed in depth in subsequent chapters. I do want you to understand the guiding principle that I live, think and write by: all of life is connected. You cannot have remarkable physical health without having a level of remarkable mental, emotional, spiritual, relational and even financial health. We are one unit and every part affects the others. However, in order to rise up a level in any one area, you do have to concentrate on that area.

There are two important areas that affect our health that I will not go into in this manual. The reason for this is these two areas are sensitive and really need a professional's help to guide you through them. These areas are often the areas that inhibit weight loss, especially in women. I often tell my clients if you are doing everything correctly to get your body into fat burning mode, and you still aren't losing weight, then look at these two things; toxicity and hormones. There are some simple things I will suggest to detox your body, but a heavy detox and the chelation of metals and other things needs to be done under the guidance of a professional. Likewise, hormone imbalance can be a difficult thing for many. Your hormone levels need to be tested and the results gone over with a health professional. Detoxing will help for sure, but again, a professional's help is needed to diagnose and treat hormone imbalance. As you might guess, I would recommend seeing a naturopathic doctor (ND) or a doctor of osteopathic medicine (DO). Standard hormone treatment with a doctor (MD) usually doesn't investigate the underlying problems, nor does it seek a natural remedy. Working naturally with your body is much better than putting more foreign chemicals into your body in nearly every case.

Elevation

I look at life like a stairway. Every step leads you either higher or lower, otherwise you are marching in place. When I talk about elevating to the next level of physical health, I am talking about elevating the way you operate your life, which in turn will produce the lifelong results you want. Take your finances for instance. If your finances are in an unknown state or bad, your first level is to understand just how bad it is and why. You have to perform a financial assessment. Then you can get a handle on what you are spending and what your necessary expenses are every month. The next level is to set up a spending plan. The next level is to spend only what you have planned. I think you get the point. Believe it or not, there are many levels to be attained within the realm of finances, just as there are in physical health.

Starting Blocks

Your starting place is different than everyone else. You are not anyone else, you are you, so start with where you are. You may have been dealt a tough hand growing up or had severe emotional trauma, or a terrible and debilitating disease. You can overcome it. You are nobody's victim and are destined to be remarkable in every area of your life. You may be severely out of shape, overweight, or you may be skinny and fit but have a horrible diet. Your body may look fantastic, but you rarely rest and are on the go all the time. You may be able to run a six minute mile or not even run an entire mile. Wherever you are, start there and elevate your health. Don't settle for mediocre – plan for, dream of, strive towards and believe for greatness.

Other Tools

When you are working with wood, you need various tools to be a successful wood worker. The purpose of this manual is to give you some tools. There are other tools that have tremendous benefit such as my book, Total Life Pursuit, as well as my website (totallifepursuit.org) where you will find exercises needed for great health, proper nutrition, lifestyle eating, and the other resources that will bring about remarkable health along with plenty of encouragement. There are so many tools out there that can help you develop your understanding and encourage you toward greater health. You just have to dig a little and you will find software, apps and plenty of websites that are dedicated to health and fitness. (One of my favorites is Dr. Mercola). I encourage you to search and find things that will help you stay focused, informed and motivated.

Crisis Attention

If you are in crisis, you may need immediate personal intervention. You may need some help and we are here to give it to you and guide you in a direction of the help you need. If you are on the verge of a mental breakdown, emotional breakdown, marital breakdown, physical breakdown or any other type of breakdown, it will affect every other part of your life including your relationship with God. If you need help in any of those areas, I implore you to seek help. Call your mentor or a trusted friend, see a counselor, hire a health coach or go to a good holistic doctor. Whatever you do, if you are in crisis, don't go through it alone. Maybe you have some profound health difficulties. This section of the manual will help, however you may need more than just this tool.

Disclaimers

Disclaimer #1: Before you change your eating habits or start any exercise program, you should check with your doctor first. This is especially true for those who are currently under a doctor's care for any disease or malady, those who take prescription medication, or for those who are severely out of shape or overweight.

Disclaimer #2: Some of you have attained a level of eating or fitness that will be beyond what I am recommending. If you are eating organically or your fitness routine includes riding 25 miles or more 5 days per week (or an equivalent level of fitness), then some of the goals are not going to be very challenging. My encouragement to you is to challenge yourself! Write in your own goals and complete the goals that apply to your level listed below. Start where you are and move upward. If you need help with a challenge and setting upward goals, email me (totallifepursuit@gmail.com) and I will be happy to help you.

Week 1

The written portion of this manual is designed to be completed in approximately 20 minutes per day. There is more time involved when you count exercising and developing a healthy eating lifestyle. If you want to raise your level of health and fitness, you are going to have to spend time doing it. Go for it!

Your week 1 assignments are:
- Complete the "What Are You Eating?" section
- Complete the "Finding Your Motivation" section
- Work on "Self-Discovery Part 1"
- Move your body for 20 minutes per day for 3 days. It doesn't matter if it is walking or working out. Just move.

What Are You Eating?

Enter your eating and drinking for the next three days into an app of your choice (e.g., Cronometer (this is my favorite), Lose It, My Fitness Pal, or www.calorieking.com). Don't leave anything out. Include all your beverages and snacks you consume and record your totals each day in the chart below. Log it as you eat it or right after you eat it rather than recapping at the end of the day. Add up your 3-Day Total, then divide it by 3 and record it in the second chart below to find your daily averages.

DAILY TOTALS:	Day 1	Day 2	Day 3	3-Day Total
Calories				
Proteins				
Carbohydrates				
Fats				

RESULTS:	Average Calories	Average Proteins	Average Carbohydrates	Average Fats
3-day total ÷ 3				

Go back and look at what you consumed each day. What are your thoughts on the *kind* of food you ate?

_____

_____

_____

_____

_____

_____

_____

What are your thoughts on how *much* food you ate?

_____

_____

_____

_____

What vitamins or minerals were you lacking, (if your app tracks these details)?

_____

_____

_____

_____

All of these calorie counters are not perfect. They are a tool in your tool belt. The reason I like and paid for Cronometer is because it gives you an overview of many vitamins and minerals. This is important because it can help you see any deficiencies that need to be remedied by changing your eating or supplements. Short of specific blood tests and urine testing, this is a good way of discovering any specific deficiencies.

Everyone has their thoughts on the ratio of macronutrients we need. My opinion is everyone is different! You have to find out what works for you, not what works for me or your friend. It can be very different from person to person. Also, once your body is tuned up and is the fat burning machine it was created to be, the ratio will or can change. My advice is to aim for the following balance:

Carbohydrates should stay under 60% and I would recommend them to be 35-50% of your intake.

Proteins should stay under 35% and I would recommend them to be 15-25% of your intake.

Fats should stay under 60% and I would recommend them to be 35-55% of your intake.

Finding Your Motivation

The Health Belief Model is a widely-used framework for motivating people to engage in healthy behavior based on a perceived threat of a health problem.[1] However, each person has to find their own motivation. You have to determine what is going to motivate you through the difficulties of eating well, exercising daily, sleeping enough and so on. You have to begin with the question, "Why am I doing this?" The answer will either be external or internal motivating factors. Internal motivating factors are the ones that will last.

Before we get to what motivates us, the first question may need to be, "What has *demotivated* us?"

---

[1] Jones, Christina, L., et al. "The Health Belief Model as an Explanatory Framework in Communication Research…" https:/ www.ncbi.nlm.nih.gov/pmc/articles/PMC4530978/.

What failures from past efforts have held you back from trying again in the area of physical health?

_____

_____

_____

_____

_____

_____

What have you learned or been told by others that has discouraged you from trying to get fit, lose weight, or achieve any other health goal?

_____

_____

_____

_____

_____

_____

Finding your "why" is essential for long term success. So let's explore a few things. Is there a fond memory of the "past" YOU that you want to be like again? If so, articulate it:

_____

_____

_____

_____

_____

Is there something that you would like to be in the future?

_____

_____

_____

_____

_____

Extrinsic (external) factors can play a part in your motivation especially when blended with intrinsic (internal) motivation.

Some examples of external motivating factors are:
- The doctor warns you that you need to change your diet or else.
- Your supervisor tells you that you need to get in better shape or you may lose your job.
- Your spouse says you have gained a lot of weight and need to trim down. (To say this is usually a bad idea.)

Some examples of internal motivating factors are:
- I want to feel more confident about the way I look and how I carry myself.
- I want to have more energy at the end of the day.
- I want to be able to enjoy my favorite activity.

What are your external motivating factors?

_____

_____

_____

_____

What are your internal motivating factors?

_____

_____

_____

_____

What things (not necessarily health related) are most important to you in life?

_____

_____

_____

_____

How would a healthy and fit lifestyle complement or support the things that are important to you?

_____

_____

_____

_____

What are your top 3 health goals and why?

1. _____

_____

_____

_____

_____

2. _____

_____

_____

_____

_____

3. _____

_____

_____

_____

_____

Self-Discovery Part 1

I encourage you to take your time with the following questions. These questions are meant to help you discover what you do and *why* you do it. The *why* may be deeper than the first thing that pops into your head. So often we do things because of deeply ingrained philosophies, long forgotten self-talk or wounds that we may miss. God wants you to make choices with His wisdom from a place of wholeness. Wholeness is a journey, the journey of restoring our souls. We all are on that journey. That does not mean that we can ignore the wrong thinking and behavior patterns that persist and get to where we need to be. Part of our journey is to think about and talk to God about these things. He is interested in your life!

Let's start off with a few questions. (Okay, many questions.)

I know some of these questions may be tough for you because it necessitates deep personal thinking. Getting clarity of what exactly is going on and why it is going on in our soul isn't always easy. Try to go deep and get to your underlying philosophies. There is a reason you do what you do. These questions are designed to help you find those reasons. Don't answer with what you think is correct or merely a surface answer. Think about it and involve God in the discussion. Get to the truth.

How have you chosen your exercise or movement routine, or lack thereof? What is the thought process that got you to this decision?

_____

_____

_____

_____

How do you pick the foods you are going to eat? (What is your thinking process?)

_____

_____

_____

_____

How do you decide how much to eat?

_____

_____

_____

How do you decide when to eat?

_____

_____

_____

How do you decide how much sleep you are going to get?

_____

_____

_____

Do you purposely seek enjoyment and laughter as a regular part of your life? Why or why not?

_____

_____

_____

How do you decide how much down time to get? (Include Sabbaths, relaxation, recreation, vacations...)

_____

_____

_____

What do you believe God thinks about your body? (Not your body's current state, but an overall belief).

_____

_____

_____

_____

_____

_____

_____

_____

_____

_____

_____

What are your core beliefs about your body, your health, your fitness and its place, priority and importance in your life?

_____

_____

_____

_____

_____

_____

_____

_____

_____

_____

_____

Do you take care of your body in accordance with your philosophy of the body?

_____

_____

_____

_____

_____

If not, why do you think that is? Where is the disconnect?

_____

_____

_____

_____

_____

How would you like to age physically? What does every decade look like from your 40s to your 80s?

_____

_____

_____

_____

_____

40s: _____

_____

50s: _____

_____

60s: _____

_____

70s: _____

_____

80s: _____

_____

If you walked up two flights of stairs would you be out of breath?

_____

_____

Could you sit up in your bed without the use of your arms to pull or push you up?

_____

_____

Are you sick often? _____

How often do you not feel 100% well? _____

How often would you consider it normal to get sick? _____

How many times per year would be acceptable to get sick with the flu or other virus? _____

Do you lack energy during the day?

_____

_____

When does your energy depletion begin?

_____

_____

Do you eat what your body needs (to your present understanding), or what you desire?

_____

_____

If you eat more of the food you desire than what your body needs, why *don't* you give your body what it needs? Give an example of the last time that happened.

_____

_____

_____

_____

_____

Do you consider yourself overweight? _____

Would a health professional consider you overweight? _____

On a scale from 1 to 10, (10 being great!) how would you rate your:

Overall health and fitness: _____

Health (not your shape or fitness level): _____

Physical strength: _____

Physical stamina/endurance: _____

Eating habits: _____

Balance: _____

Rest habits (including Sabbaths, small rest periods in your day, down time, recreation, relaxation and vacations: _____

Overall enjoyment of life (in general, not at this specific moment): _____

Exposure to sunshine each day (do you get at least 15 minutes?): _____

Sleeping habits: _____

Water intake (do you drink at least half your body weight in ounces?): _____

If you think you are out of shape, what life philosophy allowed you to get out of shape?

_____

_____

_____

_____

_____

_____

_____

_____

_____

If you consider yourself overweight by 25 pounds or more, what led to that extra weight? What was your attitude, thinking, or lifestyle that caused you to gain that weight? Go deep with this answer. You are looking for underlying belief systems and life practices. *Don't blame at all. Even if you went through a traumatic event like divorce, there were reasons you put on weight (like using food as a coping mechanism or simply loving food). If you let yourself off the hook and don't take responsibility, then it will be very difficult for you to make any progress.*

_____

_____

_____

_____

_____

_____

_____

_____

Do you neglect and/or overdrive your body? How? Why?

_____

_____

_____

_____

_____

_____

Do you eat when you need comfort? _____

Give an example: _____

_____

_____

Do you eat when you are stressed? _____

Give an example: _____

_____

_____

Do you eat when you are bored? _____

Give an example: _____
_____
_____

Do you eat when you are depressed or anxious? _____

Give an example: _____
_____
_____

What is your biggest tendency in relation to emotional eating (from the above four reasons: comfort, stress, boredom, or depression/anxiety)?

_____

Do you see anything that needs to be corrected in your thinking about choosing foods?

_____
_____
_____
_____

Week 2

Your week 2 assignments are:

- ☐ Complete the "PAR-Q Test"
- ☐ Complete the "Fitness Assessment #1" (you can take 2 days to complete this, if needed)
- ☐ Move your body for 20 minutes per day for 1 additional day this week
- ☐ Log what you are eating for the next three days in your app
- ☐ Work on "Self-Discovery Part 2"

DAILY TOTALS:	Day 1	Day 2	Day 3	3-Day Total
Calories				
Proteins				
Carbohydrates				
Fats				

RESULTS:	Average Calories	Average Proteins	Average Carbohydrates	Average Fats
3-day total ÷ 3				

PAR-Q Test

Physical Activity Readiness Questionnaire[2]: The health benefits of regular physical activity are clear; more people should engage in physical activity every day of the week. Participating in physical activity is very safe for most people. This questionnaire will tell you whether it is necessary for you to seek further advice from your doctor OR a qualified exercise professional before becoming more physically active.

General: Read the questions carefully and answer each one honestly: check YES or NO	Yes	No
Has your doctor ever said that you have a ☐ heart condition OR high ☐ blood pressure?	☐	☐
Do you feel pain in your chest at rest, during your daily activities, OR when you do physical activity?	☐	☐
Do you lose balance because of dizziness OR have you lost consciousness in the last 12 months? Please answer NO if your dizziness was associated with over-breathing (including during vigorous exercise).	☐	☐
Have you ever been diagnosed with another chronic medical condition (other than heart disease or high blood pressure)?	☐	☐
Are you currently taking prescribed medications for a chronic medical condition?	☐	☐
Do you currently have (or have had within the past 12 months) a bone, joint, or soft tissue (muscle, ligament, or tendon) problem that could be made worse by becoming more physically active? Please answer NO if you had a problem in the past, but it does not limit your current ability to be active.	☐	☐
Has your doctor ever said that you should only do medically supervised physical activity?		

If you have answered "Yes" to one or more of the above questions, consult your physician before engaging in physical activity. Tell your physician which questions you answered "Yes" to. After a medical evaluation, seek advice from your physician on what type of activity is suitable for your current condition.

[2] *Warburton DER, Jamnik VK, Bredin SSD, and Gledhill N on behalf of the PAR-Q+ Collaboration. The Physical Activity Readiness Questionnaire for Everyone (PAR-Q+) and Electronic Physical Activity Readiness Medical Examination (ePARmed-X+). Health & Fitness Journal of Canada 4(2):3-23, 2011. and, "Physical Activity Readiness Questionnaire," NASM, https://www.nasm.org/docs/default-source/PDF/nasm_par-q-(pdf-21k).pdf*

Occupational Questions:	Yes	No
What is your current occupation? _____		
Does your occupation require extended periods of sitting?	☐	☐
Does your occupation require extended periods of repetitive movements? (If yes, please explain.) _____ _____	☐	☐
Does your occupation require you to wear shoes with a heel (dress shoes)?	☐	☐
Does your occupation cause you anxiety (mental stress)?	☐	☐
Recreational Questions:	☐	☐
Do you partake in any recreational activities (golf, tennis, skiing, etc.)? (If yes, please explain.) _____ _____	☐	☐
Do you have any hobbies (reading, gardening, working on cars, exploring the Internet, etc.)? (If yes, please explain.) _____ _____	☐	☐
Medical Questions:		
Have you ever had any pain or injuries (ankle, knee, hip, back, shoulder, etc.)? (If yes, please explain.) _____ _____	☐	☐
Have you ever had any surgeries? (If yes, please explain.) _____ _____	☐	☐
Has a medical doctor ever diagnosed you with a chronic disease, such as coronary heart disease, coronary artery disease, hypertension (high blood pressure), high cholesterol or diabetes? (If yes, please explain.) _____ _____	☐	☐
Are you currently taking any medication? (If yes, please list.) _____	☐	☐

Fitness Assessment #1

It is important to get to a starting place with a few things before you move on. As I said before, you should always consult a physician before beginning an exercise program. That being said, the heart rate max test should *only be performed if you are in generally good health*. It taxes your cardiovascular system, as well as you muscular-skeletal system.

1. Heart Rate (HR) – There are many HRmax calculators online to try. This is an oversimplified version.

Resting Heart Rate (HRrest): _____

Estimated Heart Rate Max (HRmax): _____

Calculation: [220 – age] or if on beta blocker medication [162 – (0.7 x age)]

2. Estimated Training Zones

Zone I: _____ to _____
Calculation: [HRmax x 0.50 to 0.65]

Zone II: _____ to _____
Calculation: [HRmax x 0.65 to 0.75]

Zone III (ONLY to be used by high level clients or approved by physician): _____ to _____
Calculation: [HRmax x 0.75 to 0.90]

3. Blood Pressure (Free blood pressure machines are found in many pharmacies and grocery stores.)

Systolic: _____ Diastolic: _____

4. BMI score: _____ (Go online and find out your BMI score)

5. Circumference Measurements

Neck: _____ Chest: _____ Waist: _____ Hips: _____

Thigh: _____ Calves: _____ Biceps: _____ Forearm: _____

All measurements are to be taken at the largest circumference with the following exceptions:

	Female	Male
Chest	*measure right above the bust line (some do it directly under the breast)*	*measure on the top of the nipples*
Waist	*measure at the smallest part of the waist*	*measure an inch or two under the belly button*
Hips	*measure at the widest part of the hip bone*	*measure at the widest part of the hip bone*

6. Waist to Hip Ratio _____

Calculation: Measurement of waist / measurement of hips

The recommended male ratio is 1.0 or lower and the recommended female ratio is .8 or lower. If you are a woman and have a 34 inch waist and 42 inch hips, you have a healthy hip to waist ratio.

7. Step Test Cardio Assessment
You must be in good shape to take this test! If you are not, don't take it!

A Step Test is performed by sustaining a 2-minute intense exercise. Begin by moderately moving up to a maximum effort and then sustain that effort. The last 30 seconds will be grueling but you have got to exert the effort to tax your cardio system. Full body exercises like jumping jacks are good for this, but remember you have to be spent at the end of it. Take your heart rate as instructed above. You can use a device, but to ensure its accuracy take your heart rate manually as well. **If you feel dizzy, nauseous or think you are going to pass out – STOP!*

Beginning resting HR _____ Ending HR _____

1 min recovery HR _____ 2 min recovery HR _____ 3 min recovery HR _____

8. Movement Assessment

Push up (30 or 60 seconds): _____ push ups in _____ seconds
You may do bench push ups if you cannot do a floor push up. Correct form is necessary as is a complete repetition rather than going half way down or half way up.

Suspension rows (30 or 60 seconds): _____ rows in _____ seconds at _____ angle
A suspension trainer or TRX is a must have device for a home gym. You can do pull ups instead and if you can't do pull ups with help, use a band and write down the color of the band.

Leg lifts (60 seconds): _____ leg lifts
Instead of leg lifts you can do sit ups if you like. If you are going to do sit-ups, I would do leg lifts as well.

Sit ups (60 seconds): _____ sit ups
NOTE: Sit ups should only be done as an activity if you have perfect form. I hesitate to include it. Check the TLP website for full instructions. (totallifepursuit.org) First, do not hollow your back, it could cause back problems. Second, do not pull on your neck, it could cause neck and back problems.

Plank hold: _____ seconds

Wall squat: _____ seconds

One-leg balance: _____ seconds;
or Balance touches (if you have good balance): _____ seconds
Balance touches are when you balance on one foot and touch the foot you are balancing on with your opposite hand every 3 seconds.

9. Flexibility

Shoulders:
With your arms straight, can you raise them completely vertical above your head and touch your ears with your upper arm? _____

Can you perform this with both arms at the same time? _____

At what degree (0 being hands at your sides and 180 being straight up directly in line with your body) does your arm bend or you fail to move any higher towards 180 degrees? _____

Posterior chain:
Sitting on the floor with your legs straight, hip distance apart with your toes up (not flexed), measure how far can you reach your fingertips past your heels without bending your legs? If you can't stretch to your heels, how far from your heels are you?

Past heels in inches + _____ Before your heels in inches – _____

Self-Discovery Part 2

What choices have you made that have negatively affected your physical health?

_____

_____

_____

_____

To make progress you have to love yourself, including your physical self. What positive messages will you think and say about yourself?

Health: _____

_____

_____

Sickness: _____

_____

_____

Body weight: _____

_____

_____

Body fat: _____

_____

_____

Physical beauty: _____

_____

_____

Physical strength: _____

_____

_____

Physical stability (balance): _____

_____

_____

Physical endurance: _____

_____

_____

What do you want your level of fitness to be when you are 65? What do you want to be able to enjoy and do?

_____

_____

_____

_____

_____

How much of your resources (money and time) do you want to devote to sickness as you grow older? What do you think is acceptable?

_____

_____

_____

_____

_____

Sleep

Sleep is essential. We need it! Many people are overworked and over stimulated to the point of sleep deprivation. In a dark and quiet room, how long would it take you to fall asleep? If you are like most westerners it would take you a couple of minutes or less, which means you are sleep deprived (it should take about 10-20 minutes to fall asleep). Our bodies need to recalibrate and recover from the day. Lots of building is going on in the body as well as rest for some vital organs. How much sleep we need is hotly contested, but the people who say they feel fine on 5 hours are most likely being deceived. A sleep cycle is generally 1.5 hours and you could use up to six of them. That equals nine hours. Can't spend that much time resting your body? Then get 7.5 hours.

If your body is tuned right, it will tell you how much sleep it needs. A great test is how long does it take for you to fall asleep, as stated above. If you are one of those people who say that all you need is 3 or 4 hours, then go to a quiet room during the day and close your eyes. How long does it takes you to go to sleep? If it takes only a few minutes, you aren't sleeping enough at night. You can't cheat your sleep and not suffer the consequences. Heart disease, cancer, diabetes and other diseases are linked to lack of sleep, as are memory problems, lack of creativity, and the ability to think quickly. Who wants to be tired anyway? Get some sleep. Arrange your life to live it to the full, which usually includes at least five sleep cycles or 7.5 hours of sleep.

How much sleep do you get per night, on average? _____

What is your regular shortest night of sleep? Hours: _____ Day of the week: _____

Are you sleepy during the daytime? _____

What time do you get sleepy? _____

Could you take a quick nap at that time? _____

How long does it take you to fall asleep at night? _____

Would you describe your sleep as refreshing? _____

If you sat down and closed your eyes mid-day, how long would it take you to fall asleep? _____

Do you sleep solid through the night? _____

Do you have a bedtime routine? What is it? _____

_____

_____

_____

Does that work for you? _____

_____

_____

How many hours per night would you like to sleep? _____

Could you take a cat nap during a certain time? Which days? _____

Rest (Not Sleeping)

There is this idea that the Jews call a Sabbath. (Actually God said it first). The simple principal of the Sabbath for the body is resting. The Bible says that everything needs a rest. It is engineered into many systems of this planet and its life forms. A day off is not just a good idea, it is a necessity to living healthy and whole. I know that activity junkies may want to be in a state of thrill during their rest day, however, this too elicits an adrenal response. So let's think about real rest, something enjoyable that could be recreational but doesn't cross the line into intense thrill. With that brief introduction, let's think about the different ways you rest and enjoy life...or don't.

Do you ever take 3 minutes or so and meditate or breathe in order to relax during the day? _____
Try it right now! Set a timer for 3 minutes and just relax and breath deep. Think about God's goodness.

How many hours a week (not counting a Sabbath or sleep) do you relax? _____

How many hours a week do you devote to recreation? _____

How many hours a week do you plan some enjoyment? _____

What do you do to relax?

_____

_____

_____

_____

What do you do for enjoyment?

_____

_____

_____

_____

Do you ever take a day off from all work duties? _____ If not, why not? _____

_____

_____

_____

Do you take a vacation at least once a year? _____

Do you plan it or do you hope it happens? _____

If you see that you are lacking in rest, recreation and enjoyment, do you think you are superman or superwoman? _____ (If so, please try to fly and see how that goes. Use the couch as a landing spot so you don't get hurt).

Some people are content in working seven days a week for eight to twelve hours a day with no vacations for some weird performance issue or religious reason. Thoughtfully approach this section with an open mind to change the way you live. If you can't answer this for yourself, sit down with a good friend that doesn't have your schedule and have them help you fill it out.

Thinking about rest, recreation and enjoyment, what are some things you would like to see in your life?

_____

_____

_____

What could you do for a mid-day break (even if it is only for 3 minutes)?

_____

_____

_____

What would you like to do for recreation?

_____

_____

_____

What day of the week would you like to take totally off from work duties?

_____

_____

_____

What do you allow yourself to do on your Sabbath?

_____

_____

_____

Many times single moms and others may only have one day to get housework done. What could you do different during the week so you could create more downtime without killing yourself during the week?

_____

_____

_____

Don't give up! Sometimes things are tough and life is hard. Ask God to give you strategies to help you. He wants to help!

What kind of activities do you really enjoy?

_____

_____

_____

_____

_____

What can you do to start enjoying the small things in life?

_____

_____

_____

_____

_____

Water

Your body is about 70 percent water. Your muscles are about 75 percent water. Your brain cells are about 85 percent water. Your blood is approximately 82 percent water. Even your bones are approximately 25 percent water.[3]

How much water (not other liquids) do you consume every day? _____

What other beverages do you consume?

Beverage	Ounces	Sugars	Calories	How often?

Are any beverages you consume actually a beverage that dehydrates you? _____
(Alcohol and sodas are dehydrating beverages.)

Do you drink enough water? The generally accepted guideline for normal water consumption is half your body weight in ounces. (E.g., If you weigh 150 pounds you should consume 75 ounces of water per day.)

_____

_____

[3] Colbert, Don. *The Seven Pillars Of Health (Kindle Locations 195-199). Charisma House. Kindle Edition.*

Thinking about your total beverage consumption, what strategy would fit your lifestyle to bring your water consumption up to the recommended level for your current weight?

_____

_____

_____

According to the American College of Sports Medicine, to avoid dehydration, active people should drink at least 16 to 20 ounces of fluid one to two hours before an outdoor activity. After that, you should consume 6 to 12 ounces of fluid every 10 to 15 minutes that you are outside. When you are finished with the activity, you should drink more. How much more? In order to replace what you have lost, at least another 16 to 24 ounces (which equals 2 to 3 cups).[4]

What can you use during your activity, or at the gym, to help you stay hydrated with the proper amount of water?

_____

Sunshine

Sunshine on our skin does more than make you feel good, it makes you good inside. This is a touchy subject because we have heard for years that you will get skin cancer if you spend time in the sun. I am not saying to go outside until your skin is fried. Do not overdo it. However, you do need to get out in the sun. Our skin produces Vitamin D when we are exposed to the sun's Ultraviolet B rays. It really is quite an amazing design. All we need is 15 to 20 minutes per day on our forearms to get enough. Vitamin D is an amazing substance with a receptor in just about every cell in your body. In other words, it is essential. It is probably one of the greatest cancer fighting substances known to man. You can take it orally, but you need the right kind and you need a fair amount of it. The sun is the best provider of Vitamin D.

When is cold and flu season? It is interesting to note that it is during the season of the least amount of sun, when many only see the sun through a window because it is too cold outside to not be bundled up.

Do you get enough sunlight exposure? _____ If not, why not? _____

_____

_____

_____

What can you do to change that? Develop a strategy!

_____

_____

_____

[4] https://my.clevelandclinic.org/health/articles/avoiding-dehydration.

Touch

Michelangelo said, "To touch can be to give life." He was right. Touch heals. Touch reduces stress. Touch helps premature babies gain weight. Touch improves friendship. Touch charges the immune system. It's harder to touch in the U.S. because of our culture. An experiment was conducted and friends were observed talking at a café. In the U.S., friends touched twice an hour when exuberant. In France the number goes up to 110, and in Puerto Rico the number was 180! (I am going to Puerto Rico!) We are generally not good at touch here in the states. How about you?

Do you touch other people often? _____

Do other people touch you often? _____

Do you think most (non-sexual) touch is inappropriate between casual friends or coworkers? Why or why not?

_____

_____

Do you like to be touched? If not, why not?

_____

_____

_____

_____

If I quoted twelve studies on the benefits of touch, would that change the way you live? _____

If not, why not? What is your underlying issue?

_____

_____

_____

_____

What can you do to touch and be touched more often without crossing boundaries?

_____

_____

_____

Laughter

Laughter releases an instant flood of feel-good chemicals that boosts the immune system and almost instantly reduces your levels of stress hormones. For example, a really good belly laugh can make cortisol drop by 39% and adrenalin by 70%, while feel-good hormones (endorphins) are increased by 29%. It can even make growth hormones skyrocket by 87%! Other research shows how laughter boosts your immune system by increasing disease-fighting cells. Laughter protects your heart, because when you laugh and enjoy yourself, your body releases chemicals that improve the function of your blood vessels and increases blood flow, protecting against a heart attack. Fun reduces damaging stress chemicals quickly, which, if they hang around in your body for too long, will make you mentally and physically sick. Fun and laughter increase your energy levels. Laughing is good for the soul and the body.

Do you look for opportunities to laugh?

_____

_____

_____

What cracks you up?

_____

_____

_____

Can you laugh on purpose? _____ *(Try it. Laugh for 30 seconds.)*

Elevating to the Next Level

What do you think you need to learn in order to elevate to the level of health you want to achieve in the following physical health areas?

Exercise: _____

_____

_____

_____

Eating: _____

_____

_____

_____

Other health factors (i.e., refreshment, thinking right, gut health, sunshine, water, laughing).

_____

_____

_____

_____

_____

_____

I hope you learned and grew a lot over the past days of answering the many questions in this chapter. Remember to continue answering every question thoroughly if you haven't finished, taking your time on the questions that necessitate deep and reflective thought.

Week 3

Welcome to week three! If you answered at least 80% of those questions, congratulations! I know they are tough for many people. You have made incredible progress. Keep it going this week!

Your week 3 assignments are:
- Complete the "Personal Goals" section
- Complete "The Healthier You Plan" for this week

I have created logs for you to record your daily routines as you work "The Healthier You Plan" for these remaining four weeks. I am going to suggest certain milestones be attained for each week. If you already live this way, ask more of yourself. Every week I will give you three levels of challenges to attain each day or week. You are empowered to choose which challenge you will attain in each area. Whatever you choose, hit the target! Make the decision to do it and win the battle for it. These sheets are reproducible for personal use, so feel free to continue on well after the six weeks are completed.

Personal Goals

Take a moment and set some initial health goals.

Change = Choice + Strength + Effort

How fit do you want to be? (I want to be fit enough to: climb stairs, take walks, do sit ups, do pushups, play with my grandkids, etc.)

_____

_____

_____

How many flights of stairs would you like to climb before needing a rest? _____

How many times a year is acceptable to fight through the flu or colds? _____

How would you like to specifically change your eating habits? _____

_____

_____

_____

_____

What 2 things do you want cut from your diet?

1. _____

2. _____

What 2 things do you want to add to your diet?

1. _____

2. _____

Describe your goals for resting: _____

_____

_____

_____

How many hours of sleep would you like to get? _____

How many ounces of water do you want to drink daily? _____

How much time outside would you like to get daily? _____

List any goals for health and fitness you have in the following categories:

Stabilization – Balance and stability in all ranges of movement

_____

_____

_____

Endurance – Ability to continue in a moderate or intense exercise

_____

_____

_____

Strength – Ability to lift, push, pull, squat, sit up (include body weight and/or resistance training)

_____

_____

_____

Body weight - What is your realistic target body weight?_____

Inches you would like to measure in the following areas of your body:

Dress size _____   Hips _____   Shoulders _____

Jacket size _____   Thighs _____   Arms _____

Waist _____

The Healthier You Plan for Week 3

Directions: For each category, circle the challenge level you are willing to strive for that week. Record the required measurement for that category for each day in the chart. The first week I want you to write down everything you eat as well. Yes, you can enter it in an app, but also write it down in the Food Log.

This week, complete the Lifestyle Eating, Food Log and Fitness Training sections. Plus, choose at least 2 other categories (e.g., Sunlight and Water). You may complete more categories if you would like. Choose challenge level A, B or C for each category you complete.

WATER	Mon	Tues	Wed	Thurs	Fri	Sat	Sun
How many ounces did you consume?							

Challenge: A – 64 oz./day   B – Half your body weight in ounces/day   C – Add 16 ounces to Challenge B

SUNLIGHT	Mon	Tues	Wed	Thurs	Fri	Sat	Sun
How many minutes of sun exposure did you get?							

Challenge: A – 10 minutes   B – 15 minutes   C – 20 minutes

TOUCH	Mon	Tues	Wed	Thurs	Fri	Sat	Sun
How many hugs did you give or receive?							

Challenge: A – 5 hugs   B – 8 hugs   C – 10 hugs

SLEEP	Mon	Tues	Wed	Thurs	Fri	Sat	Sun
How much sleep did you get per night?							

Challenge: A – 5.5 hours   B – 6.5 hours   C -7.5 hours

REST	Mon	Tues	Wed	Thurs	Fri	Sat	Sun
Did you achieve your rest goal for any of these days?							

Challenge: A – Rest, play, recreate 8 hours in a row   B –10 hours in a row   C - 12 hours in a row

LAUGHTER	Mon	Tues	Wed	Thurs	Fri	Sat	Sun
How many belly laughs did you have each day?							

Challenge: A – 5 laughs   B – 8 laughs   C – 10 laughs

ENJOYMENT	Mon	Tues	Wed	Thurs	Fri	Sat	Sun
Did you reach your enjoyment goal?							

Challenge: A – 2 moments of pure enjoyment   B – 4 moments   C – 5 moments

*LIFESTYLE EATING	Mon	Tues	Wed	Thurs	Fri	Sat	Sun
Did you achieve your challenge?							

Challenge: A – No soda   B – No sugar drinks C – No juice/drinks with sugar added (Be a stud. Do all 3!)

*FOOD LOG	Breakfast	Snack	Lunch	Snack	Dinner	Snack
Monday						
Tuesday						
Wednesday						
Thursday						
Friday						
Saturday						
Sunday						

Did you learn anything by writing down and seeing the things you ate? If so, what did you learn?

_____

_____

Fitness Training

Below is your exercise log. You can find workout routines on my website, totallifepursuit.org. There are plenty of apps and DVD's on the market as well. You get to decide! Be empowered. If you need help, refer to my website. Remember to rest your muscles that you have worked for 48 hours so they can completely rebuild. After four weeks you need to change your workout routine.

If you are brand new to exercising or you haven't exercised in a while, start off slow and easy. Your body will take two to three weeks to get used to working out. Do NOT go hard. Do not lift heavy. Do not go to failure. Do not get out of breath. Your task is to get moving. After week three you may step it up a little.

***Disclaimer: Consult a doctor before beginning a workout routine and regimen. If you have any conditions or are pregnant, you should not exercise until you have seen your doctor. If you get dizzy, nauseous or on the verge of passing out – STOP! That is your body telling you that you are over doing it or that something is wrong.*

*FITNESS LOG	Mon	Tues	Wed	Thurs	Fri	Sat	Sun
Which days and for how many minutes did you work out?							

Challenge:

A – Move 3 days this week for 15 minutes

B – Move 4 days this week for 20 minutes

C – Move 5 days this week for 30 minutes; do 1 HIIT and 1 timed intense workout

The Healthier You Plan for Week 4

Complete the Lifestyle Eating, Food Log and Fitness Training sections. Plus complete the same 2 additional categories as last week (e.g., Sunlight and Water). You may complete more categories if you would like. Choose challenge level A, B or C for each category you complete.

WATER	Mon	Tues	Wed	Thurs	Fri	Sat	Sun
How many ounces did you consume?							

Challenge: A – Half body weight in ounces   B – Body weight + 16 oz   C – Body weight + 24 oz

SUNLIGHT	Mon	Tues	Wed	Thurs	Fri	Sat	Sun
How many minutes of sun exposure did you get?							

Challenge: A – 15 minutes   B – 20 minutes   C – 25 minutes

TOUCH	Mon	Tues	Wed	Thurs	Fri	Sat	Sun
How many hugs did you give or receive?							

Challenge: A – 8 hugs   B – 10 hugs   C – 12 hugs

SLEEP	Mon	Tues	Wed	Thurs	Fri	Sat	Sun
How much sleep did you get per night?							

Challenge: A – 6 hours   B – 7 hours   C -8 hours

REST	Mon	Tues	Wed	Thurs	Fri	Sat	Sun
Did you achieve your rest goal for any of these days?							

Challenge: A – Rest, play, recreate 10 hours in a row   B –12 hours in a row   C – Full day

LAUGHTER	Mon	Tues	Wed	Thurs	Fri	Sat	Sun
How many belly laughs did you have each day?							

Challenge: A – 8 laughs   B – 10 laughs   C – 12 laughs

ENJOYMENT	Mon	Tues	Wed	Thurs	Fri	Sat	Sun
Did you reach your enjoyment goal?							

Challenge: A – 4 moments of pure enjoyment   B – 6 moments   C – 7 moments

*LIFESTYLE EATING	Mon	Tues	Wed	Thurs	Fri	Sat	Sun
Did you achieve your challenge?							

Challenge:

A – No juice/drinks with sugar added, artificial sweeteners, or trans fat; 3 servings of veggies per day

B – No added sweeteners in anything, no trans fat; 4 servings of veggies per day

C – Challenge B, plus a daily whole food multi-vitamin/mineral; 5 servings of veggies per day

Food

Read *Eat This, Not That!* (on the TLP website). Find three foods you could step up at least one level.

1. _____

2. _____

3. _____

Track your food this week on an app (Lose it, My Fitness Pal, CalorieKing, Cronometer). Write down your macronutrients:

*FOOD LOG	Mon	Tues	Wed	Thurs	Fri	Sat	Sun
Calories							
Protein							
Carbs							
Fats							

Fitness Training

*FITNESS LOG:	Mon	Tues	Wed	Thurs	Fri	Sat	Sun
Which days and for how many minutes did you work out?							
What workout did you perform?							
Did you stretch each day?							

Challenge:

A – Move 3 days this week for 20 minutes; do 1 upper body workout, 1 lower body with core workout, and 1 intense workout; Stretch for 5 minutes a day

B – Move 4 days this week for 25 minutes; do 1 upper body workout, 1 lower body workout, 1 intense workout, and 1 cardio core workout; Stretch for 5 minutes a day

C – Move 5 days this week for 30 minutes; do 1 HIIT and 1 timed intense workout, 1 cardio core workout, 1 upper body workout, and 1 lower body workout; Stretch twice a day for 5 minutes

The Healthier You Plan for Week 5

Complete the Lifestyle Eating, Food Log, Calories and Fitness Training sections. Plus, choose at least 2 new categories in addition to one previous category (e.g., Touch, Sleep and Water). You may complete more categories if you would like. Choose challenge level A, B or C for each category you complete.

WATER	Mon	Tues	Wed	Thurs	Fri	Sat	Sun
How many ounces did you consume?							

Challenge:

A – Half your body weight in ounces, plus replenish ounce for ounce any dehydrating fluids you drink

B – Add 16 ounces to Challenge A

C – Add 24 ounces to Challenge A

SUNLIGHT	Mon	Tues	Wed	Thurs	Fri	Sat	Sun
How many minutes of sun exposure did you get?							

Challenge: A – 15 minutes   B – 20 minutes   C – 25 minutes

TOUCH	Mon	Tues	Wed	Thurs	Fri	Sat	Sun
Did you achieve your goal each day?							

Challenge:

A – Somehow touch everyone you talk to (high 5's, shake hands, fist bump, etc.)

B – Have at least 2 warm embraces with your spouse, parent or child

C – Give a neck rub to someone every day

SLEEP	Mon	Tues	Wed	Thurs	Fri	Sat	Sun
How much sleep did you get per night?							

Challenge: A – 6.5 hours   B – 7.5 hours   C – 8.5 hours

REST	Mon	Tues	Wed	Thurs	Fri	Sat	Sun
Did you achieve your rest goal for any of these days?							

Challenge: A – Rest, play, recreate sun up to sundown   B – 12 hours in a row   C – Full day

LAUGHTER	Mon	Tues	Wed	Thurs	Fri	Sat	Sun
How many belly laughs did you have each day?							

Challenge: A – Watch or listen to something funny for 5 minutes B – 10 minutes C – 15 minutes

ENJOYMENT	Mon	Tues	Wed	Thurs	Fri	Sat	Sun
Did you reach your enjoyment goal?							

Challenge: A – 4 moments of pure enjoyment   B – 6 moments C – 7 moments

*LIFESTYLE EATING	Mon	Tues	Wed	Thurs	Fri	Sat	Sun
Did you achieve your challenge?							

Challenge:

A – Continue with no sweeteners added, 4 servings of veggies per day, and 1 fruit

B – Continue with no sweeteners added, 5 servings of veggies per day, and 1 fruit

C – Continue with no sweeteners added, 6 servings of veggies per day, and 1 fruit

Food

Track your food this week on an app (Lose it, My Fitness Pal, CalorieKing, Cronometer). Write down your macronutrients:

*FOOD LOG:	Mon	Tues	Wed	Thurs	Fri	Sat	Sun
Calories							
Protein							
Carbs							
Fats							

Calories

Develop a baseline for calories. I am not big on calorie counting because you can eat poorly and stay within your calories. However, I want you to develop the discipline to limit yourself. There are many good calorie estimators (how many calories based on your stats, goals, activity level, etc) online. Choose three of them, enter all of your information and then take an average.

What is your daily calorie goal? _____

Using the macronutrient goals below, create a goal for each. (Or you can use your own, but stay within the limits I have already suggested previously.) Make sure your total percentages equal 100%.

Carbohydrate (35-50% recommended) goal: _____

Protein (15-25% recommended) goal: _____

Fat (35-55% recommended) goal: _____

How to arrive at your grams per macronutrient value:

- Daily carb intake (45%) x calorie goal = y / 4 = grams
- Daily protein intake (20%) x calorie goal = y / 4 = grams
- Daily fat intake (35%) x calorie goal = y / 9 = grams

(Example of protein calculation: .20 x 2000 calories = 400 calories. 400 / 4 = 100 grams.)

Did you come close to your intake goals? _____

What needs to change for you to reach your intake goals? _____

_____

_____

_____

Fitness Training

*FITNESS LOG:	Mon	Tues	Wed	Thurs	Fri	Sat	Sun
Which days and for how many minutes did you work out?							
What workout did you perform?							
Did you stretch each day?							
Did you foam roll each day?							

Challenge:

A – Move 3 days this week for 20 minutes; do 1 upper body workout, 1 lower body + core workout, and 1 intense workout; Stretch 5 minutes a day; Foam roll for 5 minutes a day

B – Move 4 days this week for 25 minutes; do 1 upper body workout, 1 lower body workout, 1 intense workout, and 1 cardio core workout; Stretch 5 minutes a day; Foam roll for 5 minutes a day

C – Move 5 days this week for 30 minutes; do 1 HIIT and 1 timed intense full body workout, 1 core strength with a core Tabata workout, 1 upper body strength workout, and 1 lower body strength workout; PNF stretch your legs with a partner (look this up if you don't know what it is); Foam roll 10 minutes each evening

The Healthier You Plan for Week 6

Complete the Lifestyle Eating, Food Log, Meal Plan and Fitness Training sections. Plus, choose at least 2 new categories in addition to two previous categories (e.g., Touch, Sleep, Sunlight and Water). You may complete more categories if you would like. Choose challenge level A, B or C for each category.

WATER	Mon	Tues	Wed	Thurs	Fri	Sat	Sun
How many ounces did you consume?							
Did you achieve the additional ounce challenge each day?							

Challenge:

A – Consume at least half your body weight in ounces for the day. Drink 24 of those ounces within 15 minutes of waking.

B – Consume at least half your body weight in ounces for the day. Drink 24 of those ounces of water within 15 minutes of waking, and drink 16 of those ounces of water at Noon.

C – Consume 1/2 your body weight in oz for the day + 24 oz. Drink 24 of those ounces of water within 15 minutes of waking, drink 16 of those ounces of water at Noon, and drink 16 of those ounces at 5:00 p.m.

SUNLIGHT	Mon	Tues	Wed	Thurs	Fri	Sat	Sun
How many minutes of sun exposure did you get?							

Challenge: A – 15 minutes   B – 20 minutes   C – 25 minutes

TOUCH	Mon	Tues	Wed	Thurs	Fri	Sat	Sun
Did you achieve your goal each day?							

Challenge:

A – Somehow touch everyone you talk to (high 5's, shake hands, fist bump, etc.)

B – Have at least 4 warm embraces with your spouse, parent, child or close friend

C – Touch your spouse for a time of at least 15 minutes uninterrupted

SLEEP	Mon	Tues	Wed	Thurs	Fri	Sat	Sun
How much sleep did you get per night?							

Challenge: A – 6.5 hours   B – 7.5 hours   C -9 hours

REST	Mon	Tues	Wed	Thurs	Fri	Sat	Sun
Did you achieve your rest goal for any of these days?							

Challenge: A – Rest, play, recreate sun up to sundown   B – Rest, play, recreate a full day

C – Rest 5 minutes in the middle of each day and do something playful for 15 minutes at a different time each day in addition to a full day of rest, play and recreate.

LAUGHTER	Mon	Tues	Wed	Thurs	Fri	Sat	Sun
How many belly laughs did you have each day?							

Challenge:

A – Make 3 people laugh

B – Read something comical for 5 minutes

C – Force 2 long belly laughs with a friend, child or spouse. (Be a stud. Do all 3!)

ENJOYMENT	Moments of enjoyment
Monday	
Tuesday	
Wednesday	
Thursday	
Friday	
Saturday	
Sunday	

Challenge:

A – Write down 5 moments of enjoyment throughout the week

B – Write down 6 moments of enjoyment throughout the week

C – Write down 7 moments of enjoyment throughout the week

*LIFESTYLE EATING	Mon	Tues	Wed	Thurs	Fri	Sat	Sun
Did you achieve your challenge?							

Challenge:

A – Check every label and if you can't pronounce it, don't consume it

B – Eat nothing out of a package this week except for whole food source products (e.g., butter is in a package). Everything must be whole food products. If a product has more than four ingredients, don't eat it.

C – Eat 100% non-GMO and 50% organic this week (depending on the season it may be hard to get organic veggies, so do the best you can). Everything you eat must be from a single food source. That means *you* can mix ingredients, but you can't buy anything that has premixed ingredients for you.

Food

Track your food this week on an app (Lose it, My Fitness Pal, CalorieKing, Cronometer). Write down your macronutrients:

*FOOD LOG:	Mon	Tues	Wed	Thurs	Fri	Sat	Sun
Calories							
Protein							
Carbs							
Fats							

Calories

Write down your target goals:

Calories: _____

Carbohydrate (35-50% recommended) goal: _____

Protein (15-25% recommended) goal: _____

Fat (35-55% recommended) goal: _____

Meal Plan

This week you are going to plan your meals. Yes, even the snacks!

*MEALS	Mon	Tues	Wed	Thurs	Fri	Sat	Sun
Breakfast							
Lunch							
Dinner							
Snacks							

Did you come close to your goals? _____

What needs to change for you to reach your goals? _____

_____

_____

Did you stick to your meal plan? _____

If not, why not?

_____

_____

_____

How can you remove obstacles in order to eat how you have planned to eat?

_____

_____

_____

_____

_____

Finally write down how you can better prepare food for yourself. Develop a plan of action that includes saving time and saving money while eating wholesome food.

_____

_____

_____

_____

_____

_____

_____

_____

_____

_____

_____

_____

_____

_____

Fitness Training

*FITNESS LOG:	Mon	Tues	Wed	Thurs	Fri	Sat	Sun
Which days and for how many minutes did you work out?							
What workout did you perform?							
Did you stretch each day?							
Did you foam roll each day?							

Challenge: A – Move 4 days this week for 20 minutes; do 1 upper body strength workout, 1 lower body interval workout, 1 intense workout, and 1 cardio core workout; Stretch 5 minutes a day; Foam roll for 10 minutes a day

Challenge B – Move 4 days this week for 30 minutes; do 1 upper body workout, 1 lower body workout, 1 intense workout, and 1 cardio core workout; Stretch 5 minutes a day; Foam roll for 10 minutes a day

Challenge C – Move 5 days this week for 40 minutes; do 1 HIIT and 1 timed intense full body workout; 1 core strength with a core Tabata workout; 1 upper body strength workout, and 1 lower body strength workout; PNF stretch your legs with a partner; Foam roll 10 minutes each evening

Conclusion

Before you move on, let me just say…nice going! Seriously, good work! You are a champion! If you are thinking you could have done better, then go back and do better when you are done with this manual. In fact, keep doing what you have been doing in the area of physical health and fitness as you work through the next area of life. Why would you stop? It is nearly a habit at this point. Drink water, eat well, exercise and all the rest of it. It is in your life now so keep it that way. For as long as you live. Then you will live longer and better, and better for longer!

Before you go, there are two more things to do. First let's check out some improvements. You may have dropped a few pounds or a size, but I think you will be amazed at your fitness progress which is overall health improvement! Next is the same assessment that you took at the beginning. Do it again and compare how far you've come. Cheers!

Fitness Assessment #2

Take it again! After 4 weeks or after 4 months. If you have been fairly consistent or better, you will be so motivated by seeing your progress. I know the body well enough that I am confident you have made some progress if you have followed this program. As I said before, you should always consult a physician before beginning an exercise program. *The heart rate max test should only be performed if you are in generally good health.* It taxes your cardiovascular system, as well as you muscular-skeletal system.

1. Heart Rate (HR) – There are many HRmax calculators online to try. This is an oversimplified version.

Resting Heart Rate (HRrest): _____

Estimated Heart Rate Max (HRmax): _____

Calculation: [220 – age] or if on beta blocker medication [162 – (0.7 x age)]

2. Estimated Training Zones

Zone I: _____ to _____
Calculation: [HRmax x 0.50 to 0.65]

Zone II: _____ to _____
Calculation: [HRmax x 0.65 to 0.75]

Zone III (ONLY to be used by high level clients or approved by physician): _____ to _____
Calculation: [HRmax x 0.75 to 0.90]

3. Blood Pressure (Free blood pressure machines are found in many pharmacies and grocery stores.)

Systolic: _____ Diastolic: _____

4. BMI score: _____ (Go online and find out your BMI score)

5. Circumference Measurements

Neck: _____ Chest: _____ Waist: _____ Hips: _____

Thigh: _____ Calves: _____ Biceps: _____ Forearm: _____

All measurements are to be taken at the largest circumference with the following exceptions:

	Female	Male
Chest	*measure right above the bust line (some do it directly under the breast)*	*measure on the top of the nipples*
Waist	*measure at the smallest part of the waist*	*measure an inch or two under the belly button*
Hips	*measure at the widest part of the hip bone*	*measure at the widest part of the hip bone*

6. Waist to Hip Ratio _____

Calculation: Measurement of waist / measurement of hips

The recommended male ratio is 1.0 or lower and the recommended female ratio is .8 or lower. If you are a woman and have a 34 inch waist and 42 inch hips, you have a healthy hip to waist ratio.

7. Step Test Cardio Assessment
You must be in good shape to take this test! If you are not, don't take it!

A Step Test is performed by sustaining a 2-minute intense exercise. Begin by moderately moving up to a maximum effort and then sustain that effort. The last 30 seconds will be grueling but you have got to exert the effort to tax your cardio system. Full body exercises like jumping jacks are good for this, but remember you have to be spent at the end of it. Take your heart rate as instructed above. You can use a device, but to ensure its accuracy take your heart rate manually as well. **If you feel dizzy, nauseous or think you are going to pass out – STOP!*

Beginning resting HR _____ Ending HR _____

1 min recovery HR _____ 2 min recovery HR _____ 3 min recovery HR _____

8. Movement Assessment

Push up (30 or 60 seconds): _____ push ups in _____ seconds
You may do bench push ups if you cannot do a floor push up. Correct form is necessary as is a complete repetition rather than going half way down or half way up.

Suspension rows (30 or 60 seconds): _____ rows in _____ seconds at _____ angle
A suspension trainer or TRX is a must have device for a home gym. You can do pull ups instead and if you can't do pull ups with help, use a band and write down the color of the band.

Leg lifts (60 seconds): _____ leg lifts
Instead of leg lifts you can do sit ups if you like. If you are going to do sit-ups, I would do leg lifts as well.

Sit ups (60 seconds): _____ sit ups
NOTE: Sit ups should only be done as an activity if you have perfect form. I hesitate to include it. Check the TLP website for full instructions. (totallifepursuit.org) First, do not hollow your back, it could cause back problems. Second, do not pull on your neck, it could cause neck and back problems.

Plank hold: _____ seconds

Wall squat: _____ seconds

One-leg balance: _____ seconds;
or Balance touches (if you have good balance): _____ seconds
Balance touches are when you balance on one foot and touch the foot you are balancing on with your opposite hand every 3 seconds.

9. Flexibility

Shoulders:
With your arms straight, can you raise them completely vertical above your head and touch your ears with your upper arm? _____

Can you perform this with both arms at the same time? _____

At what degree (0 being hands at your sides and 180 being straight up directly in line with your body) does your arm bend or you fail to move any higher towards 180 degrees? _____

Posterior chain:
Sitting on the floor with your legs straight, hip distance apart with your toes up (not flexed), measure how far can you reach your fingertips past your heels without bending your legs? If you can't stretch to your heels, how far from your heels are you?

Past heels in inches + _____ Before your heels in inches – _____

Next Level Planning

Lastly, let's look forward. What are you planning to do to maintain this level or to continue to grow. I realize the last six weeks has been like boot camp for many, but you have survived and thrived! Now let's look ahead and create more success through choice and planning.

Pillar number 1 – Input

What is your plan for the next 3 months for your intake? Create at least 4 goals or more. Be sure to include water and supplements in this plan. Also include how you are going to implement your plan.

Plans:_____

_____

_____

_____

Goal #1: _____

_____

_____

Goal #2: _____

_____

_____

Goal #3: _____

_____

_____

Goal #4: _____

_____

_____

Water: _____

Supplements: _____

_____

How: _____

_____

_____

_____

_____

Pillar number 2 – Output

What is your plan for the next 3 months for your output? How often and what will you do to become *more* fit?

Plan:_____

_____

_____

_____

_____

_____

_____

_____

_____

_____

_____

_____

_____

_____

_____

_____

_____

_____

_____

_____

_____

_____

_____

_____

_____

_____

_____

Pillar number 3 – Refreshment

What is your plan for the next 3 months for your refreshment? How will you create the right conditions to have more sleep, rest and enjoyment? Be specific and measurable with your goals.

Plan:_____

_____

_____

_____

_____

_____

_____

_____

_____

_____

_____

_____

_____

_____

_____

_____

_____

_____

_____

_____

_____

_____

_____

_____

_____

Pillar number 4 – Thinking

Although this wasn't covered in this manual, you heard in the teaching about the importance of this aspect of physical health. What two things will you implement in your daily life to rid yourself of negative and harmful thinking? How will you implement those two things so you can think the way you want to think?

Plan:_____

_____

_____

_____

_____

_____

_____

_____

_____

_____

_____

_____

_____

_____

_____

_____

_____

_____

_____

_____

_____

_____

Pillar number 5 – Gut Health

This is so vitally important and an emerging field of research. You heard what we know now and what we can practically do to improve our gut health. What will you do over the next 3 months to improve your gut health? What will that implementation look like on a daily level?

Plan:_____

_____

_____

_____

_____

_____

_____

_____

_____

_____

_____

_____

_____

_____

_____

_____

_____

_____

_____

_____

_____

_____

_____

_____

Teaching Notes

Teaching Notes

Teaching Notes

Teaching Notes

Teaching Notes

Teaching Notes

Teaching Notes

Teaching Notes

Teaching Notes

Teaching Notes

Teaching Notes

Teaching Notes

Teaching Notes

Teaching Notes

Teaching Notes

Teaching Notes

Teaching Notes

Theology of the Body

I am no theologian. You probably aren't either. We don't have to be to discover God's truths that are as clear as day. As you read, try not to argue your discoveries because of any preconceived notions. Let the Word of God speak to you. Many people think that our bodies mean little to God because of their theological viewpoint. So here is a quick theological checkup.

> "Then God saw everything that He had made, and indeed it was very good. So the evening and the morning were the sixth day." – Genesis 1:31 NKJV

God thought our bodies were pretty awesome. He still does. They are at least as good as the Grand Canyon or the Swiss Alps or the Ursa Major Constellation (home to the Big Dipper), and I would argue that our bodies are even more amazing. God created our bodies, therefore He loves our bodies.

> "...For I am the LORD who heals you." – Exodus 15:26, NKJV

In the Hebrew language, "the Lord" in this instance is a compound name, Yahweh Rophe, meaning Lord Healer, which God gave to himself. That is who He is. His name according to what He said, means *bringing healing and health*. Let that register for a moment. Yahweh calls Himself Healer. He must care about the physical body.

> "Do not be wise in your own eyes; Fear the Lord and depart from evil. It will be health to your flesh, and strength to your bones." – Proverbs 3:7-8, NKJV

> "My son, give attention to my words; Incline your ear to my sayings. Do not let them depart from your eyes; Keep them in the midst of your heart; for they are life to those who find them, and health to all their flesh." – Proverbs 4:20-22, NKJV

The emphasis in both of these verses is the health of our body. God again tells us that He cares deeply about our bodily health by telling you how to attain it. In these two scriptures health comes from fearing the Lord, which is paying attention, listening closely, and keeping His words within your heart because His words carry more weight than any other words or feelings.

There are dozens more throughout the Bible. I encourage you to find some on your own. Study the word so your opinion lines up with God's opinion. Next is a section that will help you get started with your study.

Discovering Scriptures About Health

I have included many scriptures that talk either generally or specifically about physical health or matters pertaining to physical health in this section. I think you will discover and agree that God cares about our bodies and our health, just like we do. Can you imagine the converse? You may even be surprised to see so many scriptures address the physical body. God put the impulse within us to maintain health. We may say that we don't care, but we find out we care deeply when things go wrong within our body. When you get a bad report from the doctor, you care! It is like breathing. We think little about it until we can't breathe. I have been in some pretty rough ocean surf before. I can tell you, when you are getting tumbled by the ocean and you have no idea which was way is up or when you will get your next breath, you panic. Everything within you wants to reach the surface and take a breath. What seems like an eternity is really only ten seconds but we have this mechanism inside of us that wants to be able to breathe. We must admit our great desire for physical health and fitness and practice it, so when the big wave holds us under for two minutes, we know we have trained for that and can handle it. Within every person is the desire to be healthy, fit and vibrant. God put it there.

As you read the verses every day, I encourage you to first *rewrite* them in your own words. Then expound on the meaning of the verse in its context. Next, make it *relate* to life as we know it. Lastly, *restore* this Biblical truth to your life by writing down any changes that you need to make to live it out, whether it is a physical action or your way of thinking.

Rewrite the verse.

Relate it to life.

Restore it to your life.

The verses are in no particular order, so dive in, play Bible roulette by randomly picking a verse or pick every other verse. Whatever you do, think deeply about each verse and discover what God is trying to say to you.

Scripture Journal

Genesis 1:31   Date:_____

Rewrite _____

_____

_____

Relate _____

_____

_____

_____

_____

Restore _____

_____

_____

_____

_____

Proverbs 12:18   Date:_____

Rewrite _____

_____

_____

Relate _____

_____

_____

_____

_____

Restore _____

_____

_____

_____

_____

Proverbs 15:30   Date:_____

Rewrite _____

_____

_____

Relate _____

_____

_____

_____

_____

Restore _____

_____

_____

_____

_____

Mark 11:22-24   Date:_____

Rewrite _____

_____

_____

Relate _____

_____

_____

_____

_____

Restore _____

_____

_____

_____

_____

Proverbs 18:24   Date:_____

Rewrite _____

_____

_____

Relate _____

_____

_____

_____

_____

Restore _____

_____

_____

_____

_____

Proverbs 3:7-8   Date:_____

Rewrite _____

_____

_____

Relate _____

_____

_____

_____

_____

Restore _____

_____

_____

_____

_____

Ecclesiastes 5:18   Date:_____

Rewrite _____

_____

_____

Relate _____

_____

_____

_____

_____

Restore _____

_____

_____

_____

_____

Psalm 118:24   Date:_____

Rewrite _____

_____

_____

Relate _____

_____

_____

_____

_____

Restore _____

_____

_____

_____

_____

Isaiah 35:10   Date:_____

Rewrite _____
_____
_____

Relate _____
_____
_____
_____
_____

Restore _____
_____
_____
_____
_____

Proverbs 14:30   Date:_____

Rewrite _____
_____
_____

Relate _____
_____
_____
_____
_____

Restore _____
_____
_____
_____
_____

Romans 12:1   Date:_____

Rewrite _____

_____

_____

Relate _____

_____

_____

_____

_____

Restore _____

_____

_____

_____

_____

1 Corinthians 6:19-20   Date:_____

Rewrite _____

_____

_____

Relate _____

_____

_____

_____

Restore _____

_____

_____

_____

_____

Psalm 139:14   Date:_____

Rewrite _____

_____

_____

Relate _____

_____

_____

_____

_____

Restore _____

_____

_____

_____

_____

Proverbs 3:16   Date:_____

Rewrite _____

_____

_____

Relate _____

_____

_____

_____

_____

Restore _____

_____

_____

_____

_____

Proverbs 4:20-22   Date:_____

Rewrite _____

_____

_____

Relate _____

_____

_____

_____

_____

Restore _____

_____

_____

_____

_____

Deuteronomy 6:2   Date:_____

Rewrite _____

_____

_____

Relate _____

_____

_____

_____

_____

Restore _____

_____

_____

_____

_____

Proverbs 15:4   Date:_____

Rewrite _____

_____

_____

Relate _____

_____

_____

_____

_____

Restore _____

_____

_____

_____

_____

Psalm 103:3   Date:_____

Rewrite _____

_____

_____

Relate _____

_____

_____

_____

Restore _____

_____

_____

_____

_____

Isaiah 53:3   Date:_____

Rewrite _____

_____

_____

Relate _____

_____

_____

_____

_____

Restore _____

_____

_____

_____

_____

Proverbs 13:17   Date:_____

Rewrite _____

_____

_____

Relate _____

_____

_____

_____

_____

Restore _____

_____

_____

_____

_____

Proverbs 15:30   Date:_____

Rewrite _____

_____

_____

Relate _____

_____

_____

_____

_____

Restore _____

_____

_____

_____

_____

Proverbs 16:24   Date:_____

Rewrite _____

_____

_____

Relate _____

_____

_____

_____

_____

Restore _____

_____

_____

_____

_____

3 John 2   Date:_____

Rewrite _____

_____

_____

Relate _____

_____

_____

_____

_____

Restore _____

_____

_____

_____

_____

Proverbs 17:22   Date:_____

Rewrite _____

_____

_____

Relate _____

_____

_____

_____

_____

Restore _____

_____

_____

_____

_____

1 Corinthians 10:31

Date:_____

Rewrite _____

_____

_____

Relate _____

_____

_____

_____

_____

Restore _____

_____

_____

_____

_____

1 Timothy 4:8

Date:_____

Rewrite _____

_____

_____

Relate _____

_____

_____

_____

_____

Restore _____

_____

_____

_____

_____

1 Corinthians 9:24-27   Date:_____

Rewrite _____

_____

_____

Relate _____

_____

_____

_____

_____

Restore _____

_____

_____

_____

_____

Colossians 3:17   Date:_____

Rewrite _____

_____

_____

Relate _____

_____

_____

_____

_____

Restore _____

_____

_____

_____

_____

1 Corinthians 9:27   Date:_____

Rewrite _____

_____

_____

Relate _____

_____

_____

_____

_____

Restore _____

_____

_____

_____

_____

Galatians 5:16   Date:_____

Rewrite _____

_____

_____

Relate _____

_____

_____

_____

_____

Restore _____

_____

_____

_____

_____

Titus 2:12   Date:_____

Rewrite _____

_____

_____

Relate _____

_____

_____

_____

_____

Restore _____

_____

_____

_____

_____

Psalm 145:15-16 (NLT)   Date:_____

Rewrite _____

_____

_____

Relate _____

_____

_____

_____

Restore _____

_____

_____

_____

_____

Philippians 4:8   Date:_____

Rewrite _____
_____
_____

Relate _____
_____
_____
_____
_____

Restore _____
_____
_____
_____
_____

Proverbs 31:17   Date:_____

Rewrite _____
_____
_____

Relate _____
_____
_____
_____
_____

Restore _____
_____
_____
_____
_____

1 Corinthians 6:12   Date:_____

Rewrite _____

_____

_____

Relate _____

_____

_____

_____

_____

Restore _____

_____

_____

_____

_____

Psalm 18:32-36   Date:_____

Rewrite _____

_____

_____

Relate _____

_____

_____

_____

_____

Restore _____

_____

_____

_____

_____

Proverbs 25:16   Date:_____

Rewrite _____

_____

_____

Relate _____

_____

_____

_____

_____

Restore _____

_____

_____

_____

_____

You can do it! God is with you.

Isaiah 40:29   Date:_____

Rewrite _____

_____

_____

Relate _____

_____

_____

_____

_____

Restore _____

_____

_____

_____

_____

Philippians 4:13   Date:_____

Rewrite _____

_____

_____

Relate _____

_____

_____

_____

_____

Restore _____

_____

_____

_____

_____

Psalm 34:17   Date:_____

Rewrite _____

_____

_____

Relate _____

_____

_____

_____

_____

Restore _____

_____

_____

_____

_____

Psalm 32:8   Date:_____

Rewrite _____
_____
_____

Relate _____
_____
_____
_____
_____

Restore _____
_____
_____
_____
_____

1 Corinthians 10:13   Date:_____

Rewrite _____
_____
_____

Relate _____
_____
_____
_____
_____

Restore _____
_____
_____
_____
_____

Mark 9:23   Date:_____

Rewrite _____
_____
_____

Relate _____
_____
_____
_____
_____

Restore _____
_____
_____
_____
_____

Romans 8:26   Date:_____

Rewrite _____
_____
_____

Relate _____
_____
_____
_____
_____

Restore _____
_____
_____
_____
_____

For video teaching, exercise routines and more health tips visit:

Totallifepursuit.org or *Totalfitgym.org*

You can reach us at: *totallifepursuit@gmail.com*

Check out our blog at: *totallifepursuit.org/blog*

@totallifepursuit

Total Life Pursuit

www.ingramcontent.com/pod-product-compliance
Lightning Source LLC
Chambersburg PA
CBHW081649270326
41933CB00018B/3406